My Christian Apology

Apologetics: Explained and Applied

Martin Murphy

My Christian Apology

ISBN 9780984570874

Acknowledgments

This book investigates the doctrine of Christian apologetics. The triune God is evident by revealing His glorious nature and character to His magnificent creation. I first acknowledge Him for who He is. His majesty and creative power was working in my life long before defending Him became a passion in my life.

This book came about because God used godly men to create a desire to defend the nature and character of the triune God. I am especially thankful for the late Dr. John Gerstner leading me to the genius of Jonathan Edwards' defense of the faith.

Some of my friends in the faith hold to different views of the doctrine of apologetics. I acknowledge their work as most useful in the defense of the faith. Dr. Francis Schaeffer left an example for all Christians to emulate. He was a devoted apologist who engaged in the practice of apologetics until his death. Until the time comes to meet the company of great men who defended the faith, I take pleasure in giving you my Christian apology.

Preface

Behold is a word found often in the Bible. It means to pay attention to what follows. Christians ought to pay close attention to the words found in the Bible. Behold, every word is important. Just as important, they ought to pray for discernment and understanding. The doctrine of Scripture is wide in its scope and deep in its content. It requires diligent study to discover the Excellency of God's nature and character.

One of the most neglected doctrines of the Christian religion is Christian apologetics. It is probably neglected because church leaders do not find it necessary for the good health of the church. "Feelings" have become more popular than rational inquiry. Bible doctrine has been supplanted by popular world views, especially pragmatism. Why engage in the difficult task of apologetics if someone will simply walk the aisle and join the church. Answering the tough questions before a person walks down the aisle, may keep that same person from walking up the aisle and out of the church.

There are different schools of apologetics and there are different levels of apologetics. Engaging in a debate with an atheist is very different than defending some point of biblical truth to an alleged theist. This book argues for a rational apologetic based on theological assumptions derived from Special Revelation. It is not written for elementary school students, but it is not too difficult for anyone who is able to read and study. It is simply my Christian apology.

The introduction of postmodern thought in this work sets the context for Christian apologetics in the 21st century. After the introduction this monograph has two major parts. First there is a brief analysis of the apologetics of Jonathan Edwards. The second half examines some of the great theologians in the 19th century Southern Presbyterian Church, especially the works of Dr. Francis Beattie. The final pages explain the difference between apologetics and evangelism.

Table of Contents

The Cultural Dilemma

I walked into a fast food restaurant and asked the cashier what kind of meat was on the super snicker sandwich. With a blank dumbfounded stare he said, "I don't know." No, that really didn't happen, but it could happen because incompetency is the norm rather than the exception in the American culture. We find it in every segment of our society. I can understand how a relativistic unbelieving society might fall prey to the "incompetency syndrome", but I do not understand how Christians have so easily drank from that well. Why do Christians tolerate incompetency? There may be many reasons for such behavior. Perhaps relativism has invaded the church. Maybe anti-intellectualism is the culprit. These and other factors have influenced Christians, but I believe the essence of the problem is theological.

The quest for spiritual relevance has driven evangelicalism deeper and deeper in pietism and mysticism. Equality has replaced equity. Ethics are determined by a sliding scale according to the non-rules of relativism, rather than the rules given by the Lord God omnipotent. More often than not professing Christians avoid the study of Christian apologetics. Why? There are too many reasons to elaborate in this monograph. One reason is the abuse, misuse, and retreat from theological studies. Another reason is that Christians do not have a theological foundation to stand on. Then stealthily the postmodern concept dismantled the modern mind.

The American culture began to adopt the postmodern concept during the last quarter of the twentieth century. The postmodern concept leaves behind all the plans and hopes of modernity. Ironic as it may seem modernity was supposed to have left behind the antiquated concepts and ideas of the past. The postmodern concept allegedly redefines literature, art, philosophy, education, architecture, fiction, cultural and literary criticism, and other cultural disciplines. The shift from the modern to the postmodern has created philosophical skepticism in the academy and practical skepticism in the public square.

In the face of modernity's failure we find the emergence of the postmodern world. Alasdair McIntyre is a moral philosopher who brought the pendulum swing to our attention long before many others. In his book, *After Virtue*, he wrote, "the enlightenment project failed." He is right in one sense of the word and wrong in the other. The failure of modern science and all its relatives has failed to give ultimate purpose to a secular world. However, I argue that modernity did not fail, because it has created another monster. It did produce something, even though we may not like the production. The alleged failure of modernity has given rise to the postmodern. The modern man was driven to the edge of the precipice. However, instead of jumping off the cliff to find some relief, the postmodern simply emerged and refused to believe that there was a death trap at the bottom of the canyon. The postmodernist wants to reshape all the ideas that drove him to the edge.

The postmodern culture will have nothing to do with the alleged absolutes of modernity. I suppose I have to say a few more words about modernity to bring my argument into focus. Modernity is more a concept than a period of time. The fourteenth century scholastics spoke of the *via moderna*, translated the *modern way*, long before the eighteenth century enlightenment. Yet there is a sense in which I agree with some scholars who believe that modernity raged from the storming of the Bastille to the fall of the Berlin wall. Modernity is the monster produced by the forces of its age such as hedonism, narcissism, pragmatism, and especially utilitarianism. Now we hear philosophers talking about "the emptiness of the modern mind" because modernity failed to meet those world and life views with answers that satisfied the soul of the culture. If urbanization, capitalism and technology, especially technology, failed to shape the culture then the postmodernist would assume that modernity failed. The blighted hope of the modern failure finds comfort, strange as that may seem, in the postmodern culture.

It has been said that culture is relative to people and circumstances. Opening the doors to cultural relativity was the beginning of the cultural wars in this country. A culture is a way of life for a designated group of people. When there is a conflict among the cultural constituents it may create a cultural war. Although we speak of these cultural wars in terms of the mid-twentieth century, they have always visited us in one form or the other. They are the battles fought over the family, art, education, law, politics, and interpretative theory. These cultural wars are fought over authority and control. Where there is a question of authority, neutrality will never be found. The ugly head of skepticism will polarize the culture. We never have been - nor will we ever be - nor should we be - free from debates in the public arena. The polarization of society demands intelligent discourse to resolve division when two parties maintain different sentiments. You may call the process of this discovery debate or disputation. It is never wise to concede to the old pseudo-peace slogan – "let's agree to disagree." However, the debates need a solid foundation, because real debates are concerned only about reality.

The dominance of cultural wars and the pseudo-intellectual philosophical debates are instruments that will lead us into a new cultural milieu. I call it skeptical neutrality. The equivalent to neutrality in physics is philosophical nothingness. If that is true, rationality, logic, and truth are obsolete. Skeptical neutrality is equivalent to agnosticism expressed in terms of "I just don't know what to believe? Is truth that important?"

Individual expressions of truth to the postmodern mind are simply nonsensical. I contend that the American culture has drunk deeply in the streams of postmodernity over the past 30 to 40 years. The axiom for the postmodern concept is the rejection of absolute truth. The result is we have a truth neutral culture. There is no metaphysic and neutrality has been crowned king. The result is the invasion of skepticism in the entire cultural milieu. Christians tried to develop a "Christian sub-culture" to avoid the hard work of defending the faith. It is time for My Christian Apology.

What is an Apology

I apologize for my belief in God and the Christian religion in the classical sense. My Christian apology is based on the rational logical truth of antiquity. I call as my first witness Jonathan Edwards, the practical apologist during the 18th century. My second witness will be the Southern Presbyterian Church of the 19th century.

We live in the age of technology and specialization. It only takes minutes to send a document to other regions of this globe with the use of a FAX, email or some other modern technology. All sorts of sophisticated equipment are available along with men and women who have specialized in a particular field. The church also has specialists. There are systematic theologians, biblical theologians, philologists, and apologists. Each one has a specific interest in the theological realm. Jonathan Edwards had a specific interest in apologetics, not because he was interested in a technical field, but rather it was part of his theology. A proper understanding of apologetics is necessary for Christians to be effective in this specialized world.

The word apologetics and the word apology come from the same root word, but we use the word apology most often in a colloquial way in the English language. For instance, Adam may say to Eve, "I'm sorry" and call that an apology. That is not the classical meaning of an apology. An apology is a spoken or written defense of what appears to others to be wrong or improper. As a theological discipline an apology is a spoken or written defense either positively or negatively for the Christian religion. The Christian apologist is one who answers charges made against Christianity by an atheist or any other pagan religion. This type of apologetics is referred to as negative apologetics. The Christian who offers proof that God exists is called a positive apologist. Jonathan Edwards was a negative and positive apologist. He was aware that apologetics was part of the Christian experience. No doubt Edwards would agree with the Christian writer who said: "Christian apologetics is not the same thing as evangelism, nor should it ever take the place of evangelism. . . .But this does not mean that apologetics is optional or unnecessary. Properly construed, apologetics is ancillary to evangelism and is unavoidable in effective proclamation of the Gospel."[1] When Paul was defending the gospel before King Agrippa he said: "The king is familiar with these things and I can speak freely to him. I am convinced that none of this has escaped his notice, because it was not done in a

---

[1] Harold Netland, "Apologetics, Worldviews, and the Problem of Neutral Criteria," Trinity Journal, (1991): p. 58

corner" (Acts 26:26). Neither did Jonathan Edwards hide in a corner to defend the gospel. He was aware that Christianity was not hidden in a corner and he could not hide his apologetics.

Christians are the only people that God calls to defend the faith. I am convinced that most Christians think professional theologians and philosophers are the only ones qualified for the task of apologetics. The Christian enterprise of apologetics is not merely an academic and intellectual process. A Christian apologist is one who sees the apologetical enterprise as a significant part of his world and life view. The theory of knowledge is inseparable from the practice of apologetics. Paul told the Philippian Christians to do the things they "learned and received and heard and saw" in Paul. Apologetics is necessarily connected with ones thinking and learning process, therefore it will require work and effort to learn how to defend the faith. The practice of apologetics, like any other Christian discipline, has different levels of discipleship qualifications.

The Christian apologist may find someone who believes that there is a god, but is not the triune God of Christianity. In another case a person may not believe that God exists, so the starting point is to prove theism. The logical progression is to lead someone to a clearer, **but never fully clear**, understanding of the nature and character of God. Many people will have questions about the gospel message. The Christian apologist must meet the seeker at his own level. *Apologetics cannot and will not save anyone.* The powerful work of the Holy Spirit can and will change the heart.

Communicating Apologetics

The engagement of apologetics must include human discourse. Hermeneutics will, by necessity, enter into the process of human discourse. Hermeneutics involves the principles of interpretation. There cannot be intelligent communication, unless there is an interpretive process taking place. Jonathan Edwards had the unique ability to employ the sound principles commonly used by the church doctors to engage in intelligible human discourse.

Intelligent communication is almost bankrupt in the postmodern world. The world has, since the Fall of man, had a problem with intelligent communication. Sophistry was introduced as a philosophical discipline during the 5th century B.C. Sophistry was a subtle false argument; it still is in the 21st century. To sophisticate means to mislead by deception and false arguments. To be sophisticated is actually bad, although a new meaning is that a sophisticated person is worldly wise, they are in the know, and on top of things. The art of sophistry is not an intellectual discipline. Oddly enough, many professing intellectuals use sophistry as a means of communication. Medieval Scholasticism contributed a new twist to intelligent communication. William of Ockham popularized nominalism. This concept denigrates the meaning of words by holding that universals exist only in the human mind. The enemies of intelligent human discourse have been many and emerge often in history.

The law of non-contradiction, the law of causality, and the basic reliability of sense perception are three components necessary to communicate truth. They are essential to the interpretative process and these principles must be used to formulate a sound apologetic. I remember asking the Edwardsian scholar, Dr. John Gerstner, what should be my top priority in theological inquiry and he quickly replied "it must be the study of the logic of language."

The first law necessary for intelligent discourse is the law of non-contradiction. Jonathan Edwards expressed his understanding of the law of non-contradiction throughout his writings in theology and philosophy. One of his most explicit statements on contradiction is found in his argument that nothing cannot exist.

> It puts the mind into mere convulsion and confusion to endeavor to think of such a state, and it contradicts the very nature of the soul to think that it should be; and it is the greatest contradiction, and the aggregate of all contradictions, to say that there should not be. . . .And 'tis a more palpable contradiction still to say that there must be being

somewhere, and not otherwise; for the words 'absolute nothing' and 'where' contradict each other.[2]

The best argument for the certainty for the law of non-contradiction is the ontological argument. God is the source of being and as such He cannot be confused about Himself. God is not in heaven wringing His hands wondering if He is truthful and therefore trustworthy or a liar and therefore undependable. The law of non-contradiction is a necessary condition for interpreting human discourse.

The law of causality is another necessary principle for intelligent discourse. It is virtually impossible to interpret rational communication without engaging this principle. In a lecture to Reformed Theological Seminary Dr. John Gerstner quotes Edwards from *Freedom of the Will*:

> We ascend and prove a posteriori or from effects that there must be an eternal cause and then secondly prove by argumentation not intuition that this being must be necessarily existing. Thirdly from the proved necessity of his existence we may

---

[2] Jonathan Edwards, The Works of Jonathan Edwards, gen. ed. Perry Miller, succeeded in 1963 by John E. Smith, 9 vols. (New Haven: Yale University Press, 1980), vol. 6: *Scientific and Philosophical Writings*, edited by Wallace Anderson.

descend and prove many of his perfections a priori."[3]

Dr. Gerstner goes on to say that "his [Edwards] whole case is to show that no action in providence can be truly voluntary unless it is caused."[4] Without causality there can be no intelligent discourse. Jonathan Edwards was one the greatest preachers to grace the American scene. The question has often been asked: "What made him such a great preacher?" Of the many elements that Edwards investigated, one is certainly the field of hermeneutics, which is a logical exercise in human discourse. Perhaps "logical causality" is the proper term. Dr. Samuel Logan, a professor at Westminster Seminary, says "hermeneutics in early Puritan thought was almost exclusively a logical exercise. . . .Just as ontology determines hermeneutics, hermeneutics determines homiletics. That is, an individual's hermeneutical methodology - the way in which he conceives of and carries out his task as interpreter - this

---

[3] John Gerstner, Lecture on the Natural Theology of Jonathan Edwards. A Cassette recording of the lecture at Reformed Theological Seminary in Jackson, Mississippi.

[4] John H. Gerstner, *The Rational Biblical Theology of Jonathan Edwards*, vol. 2, (Berea Publications: Powhatan, Virginia and Ligionier Ministries: Orlando, Florida, 1992) p. 295.

establishes the form and the style of the sermons which he preaches."[5]

The basic reliability of sense perception is a non-negotiable in the communicative and interpretative process. Jonathan Edwards has a definitive statement under the heading of "The insufficiency of reason as substitute for revelation." He posits,

> ...that the sensible world has no existence, but only in the mind, then the sensories themselves, or the organs of sense, by which sensible ideas are let into the mind, have no existence but only in the mind; and those organs of sense have no existence, but what is conveyed into the mind by themselves; for they are a part of the sensible world.[6]

John Gerstner makes the point that "the general principle being established - that most of what is learned is deduced from general propositions. . . ."[7] Edwards made use of sense experience so he would be able to communicate to his brethren in the fallen human race.

---

[5] Samuel T. Logan, Jr., "The Hermeneutics of Jonathan Edwards," *Westminster Theological Journal*, XLIII (Fall 1980): 79-96.
[6] Jonathan Edwards, *The Works of Jonathan Edwards*, revised and corrected by Edward Hickman, vol. 2 (Edinburgh: The Banner of Truth Trust, 1988) p. 480.
[7] Gerstner, *Rational Biblical Theology*, vol. 1, p. 105.

Common Ground for Apologetics

The contribution of Jonathan Edwards in the discipline of hermeneutics is monumental and should be considered by the academic world, whether Christian or non-Christian. The age tested rules for interpreting Scripture have been obscured by postmodernity. Deconstructionism is the interpretive method of the postmodern interpreter, but the deconstructionists fail to consider the weight of Puritan thinkers and interpreters like Jonathan Edwards. It is sad that many have misinterpreted the hermeneutics of Jonathan Edwards. One Christian writer asserts: "Edwards simply assumed that every passage in the Bible held the possibility of multiple interpretations."[8] That one statement shows how illogical the interpretative process can be distorted. The tragedy in the twentieth century church is that evangelicals are not reading and studying the voluminous writings of Jonathan Edwards and other Puritan intellectuals to gain a classical perspective in interpretive theory. Hermeneutics is an important dimension to the Christian apologist, but it remains only one of the many dimensions.

---

[8] Stephen J. Stein, "The Quest for the Spiritual Sense: The Biblical Hermeneutics of Jonathan Edwards," *Harvard Theological Review* 70 (Jan/Apr 1977): p. 113.

The crucial issue facing the evangelical apologist is "common ground." In the form of a question it is: Can fallen man know God or is regeneration by the Spirit of God necessary to know God? These are critical questions that separate the various schools of apologetics! A good place to start the debate is a quote from the *Twentieth Century Encyclopedia of Religious Knowledge.*

> To an innocent mind, the works of God in nature and in providence would speak of God's essential attributes; but to perverted man no such message is conveyed. True, the image of God was not altogether blotted out in man (I.15.4) [referring to the Institutes of the Christian Religion by John Calvin], yet what remained was wretched and miserable. The faculty for perceiving God in creation and in history is not just weakened: it is lost.[9]

Jonathan Edwards would disagree with Dr. Dickie. Edwards would say that it is not possible to know God in all of his excellencies, but it would not be possible not to know God. There are two disciplines that must be considered in this argument. Edwards had much to say about both epistemology and ontology.

---

[9] *Twentieth Century Encyclopedia of Religious Knowledge*, "Dialectical Theology," by Edgar Primrose Dickie.

Epistemological common ground is where the believer and unbeliever may have some agreement. Epistemology is a technical term that refers to the study of the theory of knowledge. Epistemology inquires into the source and basis of knowledge. An epistemological summary of Edwards' thought is not possible in this brief survey, because he investigated the theory of knowledge in such a thorough and comprehensive manner. To make a summary statement would not do justice to his writings. However, the primary consideration here is the question of how Edwards thought apologetically about how human beings can know God. His case is presented in many places, but his great work on the *Freedom of the Will* gives a clear picture of his epistemology.

> We find a great deal of difficulty in conceiving exactly of the nature of our own souls. And notwithstanding all the progress which has been made in past and present ages, in this kind of knowledge, whereby our metaphysics, as it relates to these things, is brought to greater perfection than once it was; yet here is still work enough left for future inquiries and researches, and room for progress still to be made, for many ages and generations. But we had need to be infinitely able metaphysicians, to conceive with clearness, according to strict, proper and perfect truth, concerning the nature of the divine essence, and the

modes of the action and operation of the powers of the divine mind.[10]

It may be argued that he was addressing Christians with that comment, but he also makes a clear case that non-Christians must possess knowledge of God. In his discourse entitled "Men naturally are God's Enemies" the knowledge is evident.

> So it is with natural men towards God. They entertain very low and contemptible thoughts of God. Whatever honour and respect they may pretend, and make a show of towards God, if their practice be examined, it will show that they certainly look upon him as a Being that is but little to be regarded. The language of their hearts is 'Who is the Lord, that I should obey his voice?' Exod. v.2... .They are enemies in the natural relish of their souls. They have an inbred distaste and disrelish of God's perfections.[11]

The question is not whether God is knowable; the question is how a person knows God. The problem is that man does know God! He knows that God is sovereign, all

---

[10] Jonathan Edwards, The Works of Jonathan Edwards, gen. ed. Perry Miller, succeeded in 1963 by John E. Smith, 9 vols. (New Haven: Yale University Press, 1980), vol. 1: *Freedom of the Will*, edited by Paul Ramsey.

[11] Edwards, *The Works of Jonathan Edwards*, Hickman ed., p. 131.

powerful and will never change. Man knows God has authority and control, and man hates that authority. An unregenerate man rejects God's authority, but a man born again by the Spirit of God can know God in his "excellencies" according to Edwards, not only Edwards, but particularly the Word of God. The epistemology of Jonathan Edwards has been explained by Dr. John Gerstner as he quotes Edwards from an unpublished sermon:

> Although the faculty and powers of reason itself remain after the fall as we shall show in the next section sin had and has destructively influenced its functioning. Reason remains but sin is effecting its functioning. . . .Man is naturally a darkened and blind creature [naturally after the fall that is] his blindness chiefly consist in two things [and here he sounds almost like Calvin] his ignorance of God and his ignorance of himself. Man is naturally totally ignorant of God in his divine excellency.[12]

Dr. Gerstner goes on to say, "Edwards does not believe that man is totally ignorant of God."[13] One of the great accomplishments of Edwards was to include the theory of epistemology in his homiletics. He had the unique ability to make it a part of his teaching and

---

[12] Gerstner, RTS Lecture.
[13] Ibid.

preaching without turning it into philosophical speculation. His sermon titles alone, explicitly or implicitly, reflect his thinking about man's knowledge of God such as "Sinners in the Hands of an Angry God." Epistemology is a technical branch that deserves the same kind of attention today that Edwards gave it over 200 years ago. Edwards stresses the need to understand the epistemological process and could be outlined thus:

1. Light comes into the mind of man

2. Unregenerate man being a sinner and naturally a hater of light tries to get rid of this unwelcome light which he cannot avoid.

3. Thus he tries to bury it out of his sight.

4. This angers God who is light and He punishes man by letting him go his way in darkness.

5. Man in his hatred and under divine punishment tries to explain away that light that he has seen and suppresses.

6. God lets him go ever deeper into his self-made darkness and the most brilliant thinkers become the most darkened in understanding, the devil himself being the 'greatest blockhead of all' according to Edwards.

7. Then God gives special divine revelation.

8. Revelation is met with even greater opposition from unregenerate men because it is so much brighter light which he therefore hates more.

9. At some point, God changes the disposition of the elect from one hating the light to one loving it.

10. Then all the suppressed light comes welcome to the surface of conscious experience and expression and with it a desire for ever greater light.

11. Converted men even grow in the light of nature. They revel in the light of special revelation. They now love light - all light.

12. Then the natural revelation which was always there and always compelling but always suppressed and always denied come into free and happy acknowledgement.[14]

Apologetics can only take place if there is common ground and Edwards would insist that epistemologically there is "common ground."

Ontological common ground deals with reality as it really is. Ontology is a study and inquiry into "being." What is knowable, according to Edwards, is that being is knowable.

I do suppose there is a great absurdity, in the nature of things simply considered, in supposing that there should be no God, or in denying being in general, and supposing an eternal, absolute, universal nothing; and therefore that here would be foundation of intuitive evidence that it cannot be, and that eternal infinite most perfect Being [my emphasis] must be. . . .[15]

---

[14] Gerstner, *Rational Biblical Theology*, vol. 1, p. 84-85.

[15] Edwards, *Freedom of the Will*, Yale ed., p. 182.

Philosophers enter the apologetic arena and argue for the criteria that must be used to present a case. One will argue that inductive logic is more correct than deductive logic or vise versa. They often miss the main criteria. God must be an eternal Being! Edwards gave himself to a study of the being of God and Dr. John Gerstner has given himself to a study of Edwards. Dr. Gerstner explained the elements of the Edwardsian ontological argument.

> 1.   Something exists and nothing cannot exist because then it would be something. [Edwards wrestles with nothingness. You cannot have an idea of nothing]
> 2.   Something exists from eternity, otherwise this something which we now experience as existing would have come from nothing, from which comes nothing.
> 3.   The being which is from eternity must also be infinite, because nothing is nowhere. Being therefore is everywhere always.
> 4.   This infinite eternal being must be spiritual, because the material is finite and temporal.
> 5. This being is also personal and thus it is evident that this infinite, eternal, spiritual being is God.[16]

The apologist, Edwards, searches the metaphysical to explain the physical. The value of apologetics was, to

---

[16] Gerstner, RTS Lecture.

the mind of Edwards, exceedingly great because of the being of God. From the tone of his sermons it is evident that he did not believe that apologetics was a discipline just for church doctors and seminary professors. He wanted his parishioners to feel the urgency, so he preached the being of God. When Edwards preached on Hosea 5:15 he said "That 'tis God's manner to make men sensible of their misery and unworthiness, before he appears in his mercy and love to them."[17] The implication throughout this sermon is that man knows God, either the wrath of God or the love of God. Edwards had "common ground" and presented his case epistemologically and ontologically. Let us go and do likewise.

---

[17] Edwards, *The Works of Jonathan Edwards*, Hickman ed., vol. II, p. 830.

A Reasonable Apologetic

There is never any presumption in the preaching of Jonathan Edwards. He cuts the fluff and puff and gives "reasons" for his faith. Apologetics is part of the Christian world and life view. Like former President George Bush said, "we can't be on both sides at the same time." Reformed apologetics is not "faith and reason" or "reason and faith," but "reasons for faith." Edwards offered many of them and to that I now turn.

Three of Edwards' favorite words must have been proof [or prove], reason, and evidence. They are used often throughout his sermons and his other writings. The task of the apologist is to hold "forth evidence from whence a thing may be argued and proved to be true."[18] The classical view of apologetics is wrapped up in those few words. The history of the evangelical church has not known any other until recent history. One of the marks of the apologists in the early Christian church was martyrdom. Men died to defend the faith, not subjectively, but with proof unto death. Edwards has given us a definitive statement. "In M 1154 Edwards wrote: 'God cannot discern evidence where there is none. If God knows things without

---

[18] Edwards, *Religious Affections*, Yale ed., p. 231

evidence, then they are evident without evidence. If they are evident to God he knows the evidence'. . . .Therefore Edwards turns to this type of reasoning. . . ."[19]   It appears that Edwards is using synonymously "evidence" and "reason." In his book, *The Freedom of the Will* Edwards gives a significant statement that is worth consideration:

> But if there be any future event, whose existence is contingent, without all necessity, the future existence of that event is absolutely without evidence. If there be any evidence of it, it must be one of these two sorts, either self-evidence, or proof; for there can be no other sort of evidence but one of these two; an evident thing must be either evident in itself, or evident in something else; that is, evident by connection with something else. . . .[20]

Speculation, theory, presupposition, hypothesis, guesswork or any other term that would lead to fideism was unacceptable in the Edwards apologetic. Fideism means to believe without any reason to believe. "Modern people like to think of themselves as independent, reasoning and acting agents"[21] according to a professor of ethics at Duke University. This presumption is not the case with most

---

[19] Gerstner, *Rational Biblical Theology*, vol. 2, p. 286.
[20] Ibid., vol. 2, p. 286-287.
[21] Stanley Hawerwas and William Willimon, *Resident Aliens*, (Nashville: Abingdon Press, 1989), p. 98

evangelical Christians. They have lost the Edwardsian apologetic which calls for logic, reason, proof, or evidence and replaced it with fideism. Jonathan Edwards followed the classical view of apologetics as a method for giving a reason for his faith. He was not only ready to answer; he made it a habit to answer questions by offering reason, proof, or evidence.

Edwards answered many questions to defend the faith like "Is there really a God?" A fair question that Edwards was ready to answer:

> As reason shows that those things which occur in the course of life, that put it to the proof whether men will prefer God to other things in practice...The things that put it to the proof whether men will prefer God to other things in practice, are the difficulties of religion, or those things which occur that make the practice of duty difficult and cross to other principals beside the love of God... .they are the proper proofs, in which it is truly determined by experience, whether men have a thorough disposition of heart to cleave to God.[22]

There is a God, because man will either cleave to God or resist God. The radical nature of man's disposition is such that he cannot avoid God. Man either loves God or

---

[22] Ibid., vol. 1, p. 414-415

he hates God, but he cannot deny God. The ontological character of God is exhibited by the metaphysical emphasis found in the sermons of Edwards. "Sinners in the hands of an angry God" clearly exhibits the metaphysical character in the thought of Edwards. The metaphors are vivid and call attention to God who transcends time and space. The sermon describes the condition of man and character of God and when brought into human experience will shut every mouth. Is there a God? In an exposition of the natural theology of Jonathan Edwards, Dr. John Gerstner posits:

> If evidence is forth coming it is incapable of not knowing God and the evidence for God is, according to Edwards, so overwhelming that man's reason is not so corrupt that it fails to see Him (that is to see His existence, not as I said before His excellence, but His sheer being).[23]

Edwards affirms that the incommunicable attributes of God do prove that God does exist. The truth of God's being is indivisible from reality. The church has lost its savor to investigate the question: Is there a God? To investigate God means that one has to investigate the metaphysical and the theological realm. Today churchmen

---

[23] Gerstner, RTS Lecture.

want to investigate the physical and the anthropological. Edwards asserts:

> 'Tis by metaphysical arguments only we are able to prove, that the rational soul is not corporeal. . . .The arguments by which we prove the being of God. . .so as to shew their clear and demonstrative evidence, must be metaphysically treated.[24]

[24] Gerstner, *Rational Biblical Theology*, vol. 2, p. 8.

Questions about the Bible and Miracles

A question often asked in apologetics is, "how accurate is the Bible?" Paul the apostle wrote, "It is right for me to feel this way about all of you, since I have you in my heart; for whether I am in chains or defending and confirming the gospel, all of you share in God's grace with me" (Philippians 1:7). The Bible is self evident because the inspired writers made claims of receiving direct revelation from God for the purpose of "defending the gospel." The notion of self evidence is present to the mind of Edwards.

> The truth now is self-evident. The being of God is evident by the Scriptures, and the Scriptures themselves are evidence of their own divine authority...It is important to remember that this self-evidence attested by Edwards is not a substitute for external evidence but a confirmation of it.[25]

Edwards defended natural theology as a proof for the existence for God. All it proves is that man will be damned eternally by an all knowing, all wise, and all powerful God. Special Revelation is the only way that man can be pointed to the Excellencies of God in the salvation

---

[25] John H. Gerstner, "An Outline of the Apologetics of Jonathan Edwards," *Bibliotheca Sacra*, (Oct/Dec. 1976) : p. 297.

of man.   In addressing postmodernism and literature, Steven Conner has said that "the ontological character of the postmodernist novel is shown in its concern with the making of autonomous worlds." He goes on to say that "the worlds summoned up by literary texts are grounded simply in their own textual mechanisms. . . ."[26] I quote him because that is the mood of the day which, I believe, is exactly the opposite of Edwards' view on revelation. Connor can make no claim for truth because truth cannot be defined except for deconstructing the text.   That leads in a vicious circle of subjectivity, but that is the inclination of many scholars of divinity at this time. Dr. Gerstner has characterized the necessity of Special Revelation as a necessity necessarily. In his sermon "The Justice of God in the Damnation of Sinners," Edwards brings us to understand the justice of God, because it reveals God to us. If then, God reveals His wrath and damnation to us in natural revelation, then He must by necessity reveal Himself to us in Special Revelation to save His people. Edwards preached a sermon entitled "The Warnings of Scripture are in the Best Manner Adapted to the Awakening and Conversion of Sinners" which clearly teaches his view about the authority of Scripture. He said

---

[26] Steven Conner, *Postmodernist Culture*, (Cambridge, Mass.: Basil Blackwell Inc., 1990), p. 125.

"The warnings of God's word are more fitted to obtain the ends of awakening sinners, and bringing them to repentance, than the rising of one from the dead to warn them."[27] The very nature of Edwards' sermons indicate his beliefs about the necessity of Special Revelation. Again, Edwards would not have to answer the question, how reliable is the Bible? He would put it in the indicative and offer proofs for the validity of Scripture.

Apologetics will raise questions such as, "do you believe in miracles?" Dr. Ronald Nash in his text book on apologetics devoted a considerable portion to deal with that question.[28] It would be proper to presume that miracles play an important part in the task of apologetics. Not only were miracles important to Edwards, they were necessary because God did exist. Edwards preached "when God told the wise and holy men to write the Bible He gave'em power to work great MIRACLES, to convince men that it was His work."[29] It is evident that Edwards placed great emphasis on the necessity to believe the miracles of the Holy Scripture. He believed that "Miracles. . .are proof of

---

[27] Edwards, *The Works of Jonathan Edwards*, Hickman ed., vol. 2, p. 68.

[28] Ronald H. Nash, *Faith and Reason*, (Grand Rapids: Zondervan Publishing Co., 1988) p. 225-272.

[29] Gerstner, *Rational Biblical Theology*, vol. 1, p. 242.

revelation."[30] It is worthy to note that miracles have been recognized by the enemies of Christianity. Edwards preached a sermon on Isaiah 51:8 and said that some of the enemies of Christianity "never denies the facts recorded of Christ and his apostles in the New Testaments, the miracles that they wrought and the like, but allowed'em. They lived too near the times wherein these miracles were wrought to deny'em, for they were so publicly done. . . ."[31] Even though miracles were important to attest revelation, they are no longer operative in the same sense that they were until the end of the apostolic time. Edwards believed that "miracles ceased with the apostolic age."[32] Edwards leaves us with the essential message that miracles are proofs and proofs are necessary for apologetics.

---

[30] Ibid., p. 171.
[31] Edwards, *A History of the Work of Redemption*, Yale ed. P. 388-389.
[32] Gerstner, *Rational Biblical Theology*, vol. 1, p. 134.

Practical Apologetics

Answering questions and giving proof to the difficult problems associated with Christianity is the reason that Edwards may be called "the practical apologist." His practical apologetics drove him to the depths of metaphysical inquiry. A question that was very important to Edwards and should be very important to every human being is: Is there a literal heaven and hell? This would have been a ridiculous question for Edwards, because to his mind heaven and hell were as real as he was. Edwards would be practically impractical if he said no to a literal Hell. His answer is a resounding yes! He devoted one full sermon on heaven entitled "HEAVEN IS A WORLD OF LOVE."[33]

The evangelical church faces a crisis as more and more evangelicals reject the reality of Hell. "Edwards finds much support for 'literal' hell-fire."[34] Edwards also teaches that hell is not only literal, but there are also degrees of punishment in hell. Edwards has said "The punishment and misery of wicked men in another world will be in

---

[33] Edwards, *Ethical Writings*, Yale ed., p.366-397.
[34] John H. Gerstner, *Heaven and Hell*, (Grand Rapids: Baker Book House, 1980) p. 55.

proportion to the sin that they are guilty of."[35] Edwards also teaches that "The torments of hell will be eternal."[36] Edwards was careful to defend the faith through metaphysical examination. He uses the physical only for analogies. "Jonathan Edwards has written that the joy of the coming world so much transcends the joy of this world that by comparison this will appear to the saint as a veritable hell. . . ."[37] Hell was real to the mind of Edwards and he was gifted in such a way that he could convey the reality of Hell in his powerful sermons.

Edwards was a practical apologist in his world and life view, but his apologetics especially stood out in his sermons. Edwards's sermons consist in the form of classical rhetoric. Such a sermon includes an introduction, explication, proposition, argument, and conclusion. Even though Edwards followed this practice, more or less, he did give a major portion of his sermon to the argument. This method permits the preacher to engage in apologetics by engaging in debate with the congregation. The debate is grounded in the Word of God, so the argument is "reason" or "proof" from the Word of God itself. Edwards obviously prepared his sermons by deduction and the truths deduced

---

[35] Ibid., p. 61.

[36] Ibid., p. 73

[37] John H. Gerstner, *Reasons for Faith*, (Grand Rapids: Baker Book House, 1967), p. 176.

are seen to be true by syllogisms. Edwards followed this pattern because he followed the basic laws of human discourse. The goal of his preaching was to make revealed truth reasonable truth to his congregation.

The twentieth century church has lost touch with practical apologetics, because they have lost touch with the practical apologists. The challenge to the church is to return to the classics. Let us remember the words of Dr. B. B. Warfield: "The fact is, despite the richness of our apologetical literature, apologetics has been treated very much like a stepchild in the theological household." Jonathan Edwards did not treat apologetics as such, because he was a practical apologist and remains so until this day.

The loveliness of God and the love Christians have for God is enough reason to defend the faith which was "once for all delivered to the saints" (Jude 1:3). The goal is to practice practical apologetics, not scholarly apologetics.

Apologetics: 19th Century Southern Presbyterians

My inquiry into the discipline of apologetics introduced me to some prominent 19th century Southern Presbyterian theologians. Since apologetics is necessary for the good health of the church, there is wisdom in examining the teaching of godly men in the past. The discipline known as apologetics has fallen upon hard times for the contemporary church. The modern church has replaced apologetics with evangelism. "Though that apologetics may not be evangelism, it is a vital part of pre-evangelism."[38]

Positive apologetics will serve to smooth out the rough areas and make the way smooth for the spread of the gospel. The forefathers in the Southern Presbyterian Church understood the value, need, and plan, if one would be an effective apologist. It is with great passion that many Southern Presbyterian Church doctors demonstrated their apologetic skills.

An apologist is one who uses all the tools available to communicate in such a way that brings the weight of

---

[38] R. C. Sproul, John Gerstner, and Arthur Lindsley, *Classical Apologetics*, (Grand Rapids: Zondervan Publishing House, 1984), p. 21.

proof upon the head of the unbeliever. This particular discipline is in a state of disorder among Protestant churches. There is not a consensus on any foundational philosophy to direct the church. During the 19th century Southern Presbyterians maintained a sense of continuity and unanimity as Christian apologists. They were influenced by Scottish Common Sense Realism. It is particularly important to reexamine the heritage of Southern Presbyterian apologetics and try to recapture a sense of how they apprehended and defended the Christian religion.

The major work on apologetics by a Southern Presbyterian theologian was begun by Francis R. Beattie at the end of the nineteenth century. He apparently intended this to be a three volume work, but never completed volumes two and three. The first volume, *Fundamental Apologetics*, was a substantial and widely read work on apologetics, which has been out of print since the beginning of the twentieth century.

Dr. Benjamin B. Warfield wrote an introduction and stated that Dr. Beattie's work was the "first to be produced by an American Presbyterian."[39] Dr. Warfield's introductory notes describe the foundation upon which Dr.

---

[39] Francis R. Beattie, Apologetics of the Rational Vindication of Christianity, 3 vols. (Richmond: The Presbyterian Committee on publications, 1903), vol. 1; *Fundamental Apologetics*, p. 19.

Beattie built his apologetical system. "Christianity makes its appeal to right reason, and stands out among all religions, therefore, as distinctively the Apologetic religion."[40] Holy Scripture has already said what Dr. Warfield claims about the discipline of apologetics. Christians are instructed to "always be prepared to give an answer to everyone who asks you to give the reason for the hope that you have."[41] The Greek words *apologia* and *logos* describe the meaning and scope of Christian apologetics. The word *apologia* means "to defend" and *logos* refers to logic and words. Christian apologists defend the faith with logical words. Southern Presbyterian theologians used those words with vigorous passion in an attempt to vindicate Christianity in the world of religious thought.

Dr. Beattie was careful to describe why apologetics necessitates reasonableness and therefore makes Christian apologetics a reasonable process. He explained that "apologetics is not self-imposed, but arises naturally from the nature of the case."[42] This is the fundamental epistemology of Dr. Beattie. The starting point of apologetics is more related to Idealism than it is to Rationalism. Rational thought is the process that springs

---

[40] Ibid., p. 26.
[41] 1 Peter 3:15 (*New International Version*).
[42] Francis R. Beattie, *Fundamental Apologetics,* p. 41.

from the epistemological foundation. Dr. James Henley Thornwell alluded to a similar thought in his explanation of the idea of revelation. "For a revelation at all to exist there must be an intelligent being, on the one hand, adapted to receive it, and there must be, on the other hand, a process by which this same intelligent being becomes cognizant of certain facts or ideas."[43] Both of these great theologians and apologists place a high priority to the concept that apologetical ideas are as natural to the human mind as breathing is to the body. These are important concepts, because in the world of apologetics there is a great controversy over the starting point for apologetics.

The most prominent apologetical school among Reformed theologians is Presuppositional apologetics. Presuppositionalists do not allow apologetical common ground between regenerate and unregenerate man. In an unpublished paper by Dr. Richard L. Pratt Jr., a widely recognized proponent of presuppositionalism, he said that "Van Til emphasized the necessity of 'starting with' or 'presupposing' the truth of Christian theism" and he went on to explain how Van Til spoke of "the proximate starting point" which describes the sense in which "all human beings 'begin' with knowledge of themselves and the world

---

[43] James Henley Thornwell, The Collected Writings of James Henley Thornwell, 4 vols. (Carlisle: The Banner of Truth Trust, 1986), vol. 3: *Theological and Controversial*, p. 157.

around them before they acknowledge the God of creation." But then he goes on to say that "the ultimate starting point for all legitimate human reasoning [is] the self-attesting God of Scriptures."[44]   I take "the proximate starting point" to mean the place that the communication begins. Beattie's idea is that apologetics is a natural process and not a supernatural process.

The natural process begins with reason which is the common ground between Christians and non-Christians. Adam was endowed with the body and a soul and the soul was a reasoning soul.   The constitution of reason was established in the human nature and although it is not quantitatively and qualitatively like God's, it does bear resemblance to the infinite intelligence of the divine being. The Southern Presbyterian theologians were careful to place reason as the first order in apologetics.

> The pretended warfare between reason and faith has been waged   by all those who wished to make a pretext for believing unreasonably and wickedly. On the one hand, it is possible so to exalt the authority of the Church, or of theology, (as is done by Rome,) as to violate the very capacity of reason to which religion appeals.   On the other, it is exceedingly easy to give too much play to it, and

[44] Richard L. Pratt, "Common Misunderstandings of Van Til's Apologetics" (unpublished manuscript), p. 8.

admit thus the virus of Rationalism in some of its forms.[45]

Dr. Dabney feels the tension between fideism and rationalism. The Southern Presbyterian theologians of the 19th century had to be very careful in their treatment of rational apologetics, because rationalism was the prevailing thought and enemy to the church. It will become apparent that these men were not opposed to reason, but rightly saw rationalism as the enemy to classical apologetics.

Dr. Thornwell left a thorough explanation of the right use of reason to guide the expanding church. In his day as in ours it has been charged "that faith is inconsistent with reason, and that Christianity repudiates an appeal to argument. Religion, from the necessity of the case, is addressed to reason."[46] The argument began with Immanuel Kant and his *Critique of Pure Reason*. His attack against reason opened the door to fideism. The word fideism denies any knowledge of God through natural reason based on natural revelation. The only way man can know God is by faith. The discriminating Dr. Thornwell makes a careful and incisive observation. First, "(W)hen

---

[45] Robert L. Dabney, *Systematic Theology* (Carlisle: The Banner of Truth Trust, 1985), p. 138.
[46] James Henley Thornwell, *Theological and Controversial*, p. 184-185.

God speaks, faith is the highest exercise of reason."[47] Dr. Thornwell goes on to say that "reasoning is nothing but the successive steps by which we arrive at the same testimony in the original structure of our minds. . . .Reasoning is only a method of ascertaining what God teaches. . ."[48] Dr. Beattie describes reason as "the mental faculty which deals with principles and laws. These laws regulate the activity of the spiritual principle of human intelligence in the supersensible realm of pure thought."[49] Reason is the indispensable common ground upon which all men meet.

The place of reason in apologetics is necessary to establish a belief system. Dr. William Plumer has attempted "to show that man may reasonably be required to believe sufficient evidence."[50] Apologetics has as its main purpose a reasonable defense of the Christian faith. The defense is made by presenting evidence so that it may be proved to be true. According to Dr. Plumer, reason is required to establish the belief system and so make the evidence believable. That is the classical apologetical method used by the church throughout most of the history of the church.

---

[47] Ibid., 187.
[48] Francis R. Beattie, *Fundamental Apologetics*, p. 187.
[49] Francis R. Beattie, *Fundamental Apologetics*, p. 82
[50] William S. Plumer, "Man Responsible for His Belief," in Lectures on the Evidences of Christianity (New York: Robert Carter and Brothers, 1859), p. 20.

One of the marks of the apologists in the early Christian church was martyrdom. Men died to defend the faith, because their belief system was compelling by the presentation of the evidence. St. Augustine said, "there can be no question but that the amount of reason which leads us to accord this faith, whatever that amount may be, is itself anterior to faith."[51]   The apologists of the Southern Presbyterian Church agree with the great apologist of the early church.   Dr. Beattie explains the relationship of reason to the establishment of a belief system.

> Knowledge and belief are closely related. . . .If knowledge be the direct apprehension of the truth of reality of its object, belief is the indirect of mediate apprehension of its object.   If knowledge be conviction of the truth, as it shines in its own light, belief is persuasion of the truth as it is seen in the light of proper evidence.   If knowledge produces complete certainty, belief is content with probability of greater or less degree.. . Hence, belief may be defined as mental assent or conviction, founded upon evidence.   It is the persuasion, more or less assured, of the truth of anything, resting upon grounds which rationally justify that persuasion.   To believe without evidence is irrational, and to profess to believe against evidence is willful, if not absurd. . . .It thus appears that evidence is the measure of

---

[51] Gerstner, *Rational Biblical Theology*, vol. 1, p. 28.

belief, and that the stronger the evidence the firmer will be the belief. . . .Belief rests on evidence, and evidence, in turn, is a matter of knowledge, and knowledge implies a primary belief in the reliability of the faculties involved in it.[52]

Dr. Beattie's argument is that the belief system is grounded by evidence. Evidence is understood by the intellectual capacity of the mind, because the intellect has the power of reason. "Apologetics will find occasion to utilize belief, and to exhibit the **reasonable** (my emphasis) grounds of Christianity."[53] Dr. Thornwell can bring this concept into clearer focus.

As it is necessity of belief which distinguishes intelligent action from every other species of operation, and as there can be no belief without the belief of something, there must be certain primary truths involved in the very structure of the mind, which are admitted from the simple necessity of admitting them.[54]

Dr. Thornwell has identified a profound, but simple concept. No belief can exist without believing something and reason is something, therefore reason is inseparably

---

[52] Francis R. Beattie, *Fundamental Apologetics*, p. 82.
[53] Ibid., p. 108.
[54] James Henley Thornwell, *Theological and Controversial*, p. 81.

connected to the establishment of a belief system. We may turn to Dr. Dabney for a clear and compelling statement in this regard. "The dictate of reason herself, is to believe; because she sees the evidences to be reasonable.[55]

These Southern Presbyterian apologists look for evidence as the ground for their reason. They do not build a system known as evidentialism, but apologetics will not stand without evidence. Dr. Thornwell uses a rhetorical question to stimulate our thinking. "If evidence had no inherent and essential tendency to generate belief, if conviction were the arbitrary offspring of circumstances, why should we be bound to examine evidence at all?"[56] Evidence leads to proof and proof is the goal of Christian apologetics. The fact that evidence works on the mind and not merely the emotions becomes obvious in the writings of Southern Presbyterian ministers. Rev. B. M. Smith said, "if the mind be uninformed, darkened by error and blinded by prejudice, the avenues to the heart are closed."[57] The use of evidence is held forth as a light to the mind to bring an awareness of God's displeasure to the impenitent sinner. "Our duty is to walk by the light which we have. God commands us to yield to all evidence that is real in precise

---

[55] Robert L. Dabney, *Systematic Theology*, p. 144.
[56] James Henley Thornwell, *Theological and Ethical*, p. 490.
[57] B. M. Smith, "Popular Objections to Christianity," in Lectures on the Evidences of Christianity, p. 407.

proportion to its strength."[58]   Dr. Thornwell was an evidentialist, but evidentialism was not the end to his apologetical method.   However, he did use evidences within his apologetical system.   In a letter he wrote to Dr. R. J. Breckinridge, Dr. Thornwell noted that he had "succeeded in awaking a strong interest in the evidences of our religion."[59]   The use of evidence in the discipline of apologetics was fundamental to the minds of some of the giants in the Southern Presbyterian Church during the 19th century.

The use of evidence was incorporated in a coherent system that manifested itself according to the sound principles employed by church fathers throughout the centuries.   Intelligent human discourse is not possible without the employment of certain basic principles. Although I mentioned these principles previously, I want to review them in the context of the Southern Presbyterianism.   The three non-negotiables used by classical apologists are the law of non-contradiction, the law of causality, and the basic reliability of sense perception.   Now the task is to determine whether or not and to what extent Southern Presbyterian theologians employed these principles in their apologetics.

---

[58] James Henley Thornwell, *Theological and Ethical*, p. 511.
[59] B. M. Palmer, *The Life and Letters of James Henley Thornwell* (Carlisle: The Banner of Truth Trust, 1986), p. 224.

Little needs to be said about the law of non-contradiction. Aristotle defined the Law of non-contradiction as "[T]he same attribute cannot at the same time belong and not belong to the same subject in the same respect."[60] One theological giant from the Southern Presbyterian heritage will affirm this basic law.

> Among these evidences, the reason must entertain this question: whether anything asserted in revelation is inevitably contradictory with reason or some other things asserted in revelation. For if a book clearly contained such things, it would be proof it was not from God; because God, who first created our laws of reason, will not contradict Himself by teaching incompatibles in His works and word. And again: in demanding faith (always a sincere and intelligent faith,) of us in such contradictories, He would be requiring of us an impossibility.[61]

The law of non-contradiction is essential to the Christian religion as Dr. Dabney indicated in his systematic theology. This law transcends the physical, because it is absent of content. The interpretive devises of human discourse become meaningless if the law of non-

---

[60] W. D. Ross, ed. *Aristotle Selections* (New York: Scribner, 1927), p. 56.
[61] Robert L. Dabney, *Systematic Theology*, p. 141-142.

contradiction does not exist. Dr. Plumer also alludes to the importance of this law. "A proposition, admitting of but one construction, cannot be both true and false."[62] He goes on to say that "logical reasonings on moral subjects may be as fair and as conclusive as mathematical demonstrations."[63] It sounds if though they would ontologically extend the weight of the law of non-contradiction to the transcendent God that Christians worship and serve.

The law of causality is another necessary principle for intelligent human discourse. It quickly becomes apparent that the Southern Presbyterian theologians did not repudiate causality as an Aristotelian concept. Dr. Plumer believed that "the connection between cause and effect in the moral world is as close as in the physical."[64] Dr. Thornwell's lectures on the "Being of God" provide a classical statement on the law of causality from a Southern Presbyterian in the first order.

> Taking then, the law of causation as at once a law of thought and a law of existence, whenever it sets out from the real it must necessarily lead to the real. If we have effects that are real, we must find causes

---

[62] William S. Plumer, "Man Responsible for His Belief," in Lectures on the Evidences of Christianity, p. 5.
[63] Ibid.
[64] Ibid.

that are real. In the theistic argument we begin, in the first place, with beings that are real. We set out from facts which fall within the sphere of our experience. We start from the world around us. Here is being, and being in a constant state of flux and change. It is being that began. If it were necessary, it would be immutable. Whatever necessarily is, necessarily is just as it is and just what it is. . . . An infinite succession of finite and changeable objects is a contradiction. If the world began, it must have had a Maker. The conclusion is as certain as the law of causation.[65]

Dr. Thornwell is indubitably committed to the idea that the law of causality is as certain as God Himself. Causality is often relegated to the world of empiricism, but classical apologists have not treated it that way. "As in the mind, the principle of causation is a priori in its nature. On its subjective side, causality is a fundamental law of thought. This means that it does not arise in the mind from experience, but is given by the mind itself to experience."[66] This is not the incidental thought of one man. Although not Southern Presbyterian, Jonathan Edwards would certainly agree with the Southern Presbyterians. "On the whole, it is clearly manifest, that every effect has a necessary connection with its cause, or with that which is the true

---

[65] James Henley Thornwell, *Theological*, p. 57-58.
[66] Francis R. Beattie, *Fundamental Apologetics*, p. 324-325.

ground and reason of its existence."[67] The use of human language, especially biblical language, assumes the validity of causality in normal discourse by the common use of words like "therefore" or "because." The relationship between the law of causality and natural or supernatural theology cannot be denied. "Few words are needed to show the intimate relations between the true doctrine of causation and theology."[68] To the mind of these Southern Presbyterian theologians, it becomes abundantly clear that the law of causality was a non-negotiable for apologetics.

Intelligent human discourse must also rely on the basic reliability of sense perception. Sense experience is necessary for intelligent human communication.

> We believe the reports of our senses and the data of consciousness because the constitution of our nature is such that we cannot do otherwise; but when we are asked how we know that our faculties do not deceive us, we can only appeal to the moral character of Him who has wrought these laws of belief into the very texture of our frames.[69]

When Calvin argued for the actual existence of evil angels, he used the reference in John 8:44 referring to the

---

[67] Perry Miller, The Work of Jonathan Edwards, 9 vols. (New Haven: Yale University Press, 1957) vol. 1: *The Freedom of the Will*, p. 216.
[68] Robert L. Dabney, *Systematic Theology*, p. 93.
[69] James Henley Thornwell, *Theological and Ethical*, p. 157.

opponents of Christ who were physically present. In his reference to them Calvin said "the names themselves sufficiently express, not impulses or affections of minds, but rather what are called minds or spirits endowed with sense perception and understanding."[70] The fact that Calvin believed and taught that sense perception was part of the nature of man is sufficient reason to believe that the Calvinists within Southern Presbyterianism would have been aware of the validity of this concept. Dr. Dabney quickly reminds us that "[I]f no first truth is of higher source than an inference of experience, then none can be safely postulated beyond experience."[71] The operative word in the aphorism "basic reliability of sense perception" is the word "basic." Sense perception is not absolute and unlike the law of non-contradiction and the law of causality, sense perception moves from the formal and independently logical to the material and empirical realm. Dr. Beattie explains how a belief system is formed and refers to a particular "class of the grounds of belief is objective and more palpable, for it consists in certain outward facts in the world about us. By fact here, is meant some real thing, or object, in the external world."[72]

---

[70] John Calvin, *Institutes of the Christian Religion*, 2 vols. Ed. John T. McNeill (Philadelphia: The Westminster Press, 1960), p. 178.
[71] Robert L. Dabney, *Systematic Theology*, p. 80.
[72] Francis R. Beattie, *Fundamental Apologetics*, p. 103.

Southern Presbyterianism would recognize the necessity of "the basic reliability of sense perception" in their apologetical system. The wisdom of the Southern Presbyterian giants concerning apologetics ought not to be overlooked. "He, who rejects consciousness, intuition, the senses, and logical reasonings, can make no progress in knowledge, and will simply live and die a fool."[73]

Apologetics is a reasoned defense of the Christian religion. The scope of apologetics rests upon mental activity and heart activity. Therefore, the essential task of the apologist is to compellingly present evidence leading to the knowledge of God. In a lecture to Reformed Seminary Dr. John Gerstner, a noted apologist in the Presbyterian Church in America, said:

> If evidence is forth coming, it is incapable of not knowing God and the evidence for God is, according to Edwards, so overwhelming that man's reason is not so corrupt that it fails to see Him (that is to see his existence, not as I said before, His excellence, but His sheer being).[74]

The process of presenting compelling evidence is

---

[73] William S. Plumer, "Man Responsible for His Belief," in Lectures on the Evidences of Christianity, p. 6.

[74] John Gerstner, A Lecture on the Natural Theology of Jonathan Edwards, Reformed Theological Seminary.

accomplished by using the classical theistic proofs. These proofs purposely drive one to theism. An explanation of theism in this context is important.

> Theism is that doctrine concerning the origin and continued existence of the world which affirms the being and constant activity of one infinite personal God who sustains definite natural and moral relations with the world, and which presents this affirmation as the necessary and adequate explanation of the problems thereby presented for rational solution.[75]

It has been suggested that Theism is natural to man. Dr. Beattie explains that "the con-natural theistic capacity must be presupposed in man in order to render him capable of receiving and understanding any objective revelation from God."[76] Dr. Beattie believes the theistic arguments are logical.

> [They are] like the strands of a cable, rather than the links of a chain. If they be regarded merely as links in a chain, the strength of the whole is measured by the strength of the weakest link; but if they be considered to be strands. . .their argumentative force

---

[75] Francis R. Beattie, *Fundamental Apologetics*, p. 120-121.
[76] Ibid., p. 231.

is equal to the strength of all the strands when compacted into the cable.[77]

The theistic arguments known as the ontological, cosmological, and teleological proofs are commonly used by Classical apologists.

The ontological argument has been abused by fallacious inferences drawn from the Latin phrase *finitum non capax infiniti*. The phrase is often translated into English as "the finite cannot comprehend the infinite." The translation is insufficient when the ontological argument is under consideration. The background behind the phrase will help us understand its intended meaning.

> The finite is incapable of the infinite; . . .an epistemological and Christological maxim emphasized by the Reformed in debate with the Lutherans. Epistemologically it signifies the limitation of the human mind, even the mind of Christ, in the knowledge of divine things."[78]

It does not mean that God is not knowable, but it does mean that God is not knowable in His Excellencies. Dr. Beattie agrees that "a merely verbal revelation cannot

---

[77] Ibid., p. 255.
[78] Richard A. Muller, *Dictionary of Latin and Greek Theological Terms* (Grand Rapids: Baker Book House, 1985), p. 119.

communicate the knowledge of God if man has not already the idea of God in his mind."[79] The ontological argument is concerned with the idea of Being in the mind of man. "We can by no means shake ourselves free from the notion of God."[80] Dr. Beattie places the ontological argument in first place among all the theistic arguments. "We begin, consequently, with the a priori aspects of the proof, and pass on to the a posteriori. The ontological proofs will thus be considered before the teleological."[81]

The cosmological argument has to do with the order we find in creation. Dr. Thornwell did not believe it was fallacious reasoning to use the cosmological argument, but he did believe the "cosmological argument fails to give us any other conception of God than that of necessary being."[82] The cosmological argument has its foundation in the law of causality which has already been discussed in this review of Southern Presbyterian apologetics.

The teleological argument is based on the apparent order and design of the universe. Dr. Beattie states that the teleological argument is marked "by the evidences of design which abound in the world."[83] Dr. Thornwell

---

[79] Francis R. Beattie, *Fundamental Apologetics*, p. 233.
[80] Ibid., 232.
[81] Ibid., p. 258-259.
[82] James Henley Thornwell, *Theological*, p. 60.
[83] Francis R. Beattie, *Fundamental Apologetics*, p. 328.

teaches that the teleological is sufficient to "prove an intelligent cause, [but] if taken alone, fails to demonstrate the existence of an infinite Author of the universe."[84] Dr. Thornwell posits that the teleological and cosmological arguments complement each other.

> [I]n itself, therefore, it is incomplete, but when added to the cosmological which gives us a Creator - an infinite, eternal, necessary Being - we perceive that this Being is intelligent, that He is an almighty Spirit, and that the thoughts of His understanding have been from everlasting."[85]

Dr. Thornwell and Dr. Beattie apparently agree that the theistic proofs are like a "cable" (the cumulative is compelling) rather than a "chain that will break when one link is weak."

Classical apologetics has been abandoned, but not forgotten. The trend among Presbyterian and Reformed Churches during the 20th century has taken a turn from classical apologetics toward presuppositional apologetics. It must be remembered that Thornwell and Dabney lived and ministered during the golden age of Deism. When they argued against natural revelation, they did not intend to

---

[84] James Henley Thornwell, *Theological*, p. 62.
[85] Ibid., 63.

argue against natural revelation as an apologetical method. They were arguing against natural revelation as a means of salvation for those sinful Deists. They were arguing that natural revelation would not replace supernatural revelation as the basis for the evangelistic endeavor of the church. Dr. Beattie explains:

> Not a few theologians of a century ago, who had not freed themselves entirely from the philosophy of deism, adopted this explanation of religious and theistic belief. Watson is an able exponent of this view. In his writings he maintains, in an earnest way, what in a sense, is true of sinful man, that human reason cannot give him genuine religious knowledge, and that a revelation from God alone can do this.[86]

Dr. Beattie believes that the function of revelation is two fold, but that supernatural revelation is necessary to apprehend the saving excellencies taught in Scripture.

In his doctoral dissertation, Kenneth Boa analyzed four apologetic systems. There were numerous references to Francis Beattie's work on apologetics.[87] Boa's references to Beattie indicated a sense of strength in Beattie's work.

---

[86] Francis R. Beattie, *Fundamental Apologetics*, p. 222-223.

[87] Kenneth Dale Boa, *A Comparative Study of Four Christian Apologetics Systems*, (Ann Arbor: U.M.I. Dissertation Information Service, 1987), p. 19-54.

Dr. Beattie was clearly a classical apologist and his work published in 1903 was representative of the Southern Presbyterians in the 19th century. The recovery of classical apologetics will be enhanced by making the work of the great Southern Presbyterian apologist, Dr. Francis R. Beattie, available to future apologist in the Southern Presbyterian tradition as well as the church in general.

Understanding Natural Law for Apologetics

Apologetics is not an easy discipline to master because it is interconnected with various doctrines of Scripture. Since apologetics is directed toward unbelievers there must be some connection for the believer and unbeliever to agree. Christians have a wonderful opportunity to engage the unbeliever since natural law is a sacred and a secular concept.

Many Christians deny that Romans 2:14 and 15 teaches natural law. Others argue against natural law from philosophical and theological formulations. One Christian theologian seems a bit confused by asserting, "natural law is based on an unbiblical epistemology." Then he wrote:

> I affirm that, though unregenerate sinners invariably know God and certain truths about Him and His Law, and indeed may know many truths about God, special revelation challenges, confronts, and undermines their fundamentally distorted natural theologies and natural codes."[88]

The question is not whether or not there is an

---

[88] Peter Leithart, "Premise," Vol. 3, No. 2, Feb. 29, 1996.

epistemological a priori connected with the law of God. Epistemology refers to the inquiry into the source and value of knowledge. However, my concern is ontological. To put it another way does natural law exist? The quality or the quantity of natural law in reality will be the subject of another inquiry. The Bible clearly affirms natural law.

> [F]or when Gentiles, who do not have the law, by nature do the things in the law, these, although not having the law, are a law to themselves, who show the work of the law written in their hearts, their conscience also bearing witness, and between themselves their thoughts accusing or else excusing them. . .(Romans 2:14 and 15).

John Calvin makes a comment on this text that must be repeated over and over again. Calvin said: "All nations. . .have some notions of justice. . .which The Greeks call preconceptions, and which are implanted by nature in the hearts of men."[89] The New King James Version used the word "Gentiles" and Calvin used the word "nations." The Greek word *ethnos* translated into English as "Gentiles" or "nations" is a plural noun in the Romans text. Paul's emphasis in his letter to the Romans has been either on the Jews or the *ethnos* (Gentiles or nations, plural), so

---

[89] John Calvin, *Calvin's Commentaries* vol. 19 (Grand Rapids, MI. : Baker Book House,) p. 96

the word Gentile or nations represents all people groups other than the Jews. John Calvin is one among many of God's servants who believed that the Bible teaches natural law.

The rebirth of natural law in modern times has been attributed to the Roman Catholic Church. It is sad that we have to think in those terms because the church should not have to give rebirth to something that is plainly taught in Scripture. We must not think the concept of natural law was an invention of recent times. Our church fathers from the first century until now have acknowledged natural law, even if it is much despised today. Let me give you a few examples from the early history of the church.

Tertullian (160 - 215)   Time even the heathens observe, that, in obedience to the law of nature, they may render their own rights to the (different) ages. For their females they dispatch to their businesses from (the age of) twelve years, but the male from two years later; decreeing puberty (to consist) in years, not in espousals or nuptials. "Housewife" one is called, albeit a virgin, and "house-father," albeit a stripling. By us not even natural laws are observed; as if the God of nature were some other than ours! (Ante-Nicene Fathers, Volume IV, Part Fourth, On the Veiling of Virgins, Chap. 11)

St. Chrysostom (344-407)   For this reason, here dismissing this subject; and having given to the laborious and studious an opportunity, by what has been said, of going over likewise the other parts of Creation; we shall now direct our discourse to another point which is itself also demonstrative of God's providence. What then is this second point? It is, that when God formed man, he implanted within him from the beginning a natural law. And what then was this natural law? He gave utterance to conscience within us; and made the knowledge of good things, and of those that are the contrary, to be self-taught. (Concerning the Statutes, Homily 12. P. 421)

The evidence for natural law is found in great abundance, apart from Scripture.

- From the heathen world - Plato and Aristotle made explicit reference to natural law.
- From the absurdity of no law.
- From the ontological argument - Something created creation. That something was God, therefore God is in control of His creation, because dependent beings must rely on an Independent Being for any source of order, authority, power, and morality.

Natural law is found in early Greek philosophical thought, it is found in Christian theological expressions, and it is found among heathen writers who make no claim to clarify its definition.

The church of all ages has acknowledged natural law. Sometimes referred to as the law of nature, natural law has come under attack by some theologians in the contemporary church. The concept of natural law found in Romans 2:14 and 15 demands our careful attention. It is necessary to clarify the meaning of the words "natural law" in the context of Romans chapter two.

First, let me tell you what natural law is not. Natural law is not natural revelation. Natural revelation is a term used to describe what theologians call general revelation. General revelation refers to the scope and content of God making Himself known. The scope is the whole world and the content is limited to natural theology. Natural theology is a concept that refers to the knowledge people have of God through general revelation.

Natural law is so ill defined today that the term itself must be scrutinized in its context. Natural law theories seem to find a home in reason often referred to as rationality. Many theologians associate natural law with rationalism. For instance one theologian wrote:

> Natural law in Christian theology traditionally refers to the inherent and universal structures of human existence which can be discerned by the unaided reason and which form the basis for judgments of conscience about the good and evil and which therefore make it possible to say that that

right is the rational (*A Handbook of Theological Terms*, by Van A. Harvey).

It will be fruitless to examine all the definitions of natural law used in recent times. Webster's definition is: "a principle or body of laws considered as derived from nature, right reason, or religion and ethically binding in human society." If we use that definition, it would require an explication beyond the scope of this monograph. Furthermore, it would demand inquiry into every philosophical and theological reference contained in that dictionary definition. There are so many different ways to define natural law that time will not permit inquiry into all the false claims in this study. For instance, St. Thomas Aquinas denies natural law in some sense, but refers to it as eternal law. Then how do we answer Romans 2:14 Aquinas asked? Aquinas answers his rhetorical question.

> I answer that, as we have stated above, law, being a rule and measure, can be in a person in two ways: in one way, as in him that rules and measures; in another way, as in that which is ruled and measured, since a thing is ruled and measured in so far as it partakes of the rule or measure. Therefore, since all things subject to divine providence are ruled and measured by the eternal law. . ., it is evident that all things partake in some way in the eternal law, in so far as, namely from its being imprinted on them, they derive their respective inclinations to their

> proper acts and ends... . Therefore it has a share of the eternal reason, whereby it has a natural inclination to its proper act and end; and this participation of the eternal law in the rational creatures is called the natural law.[90]

For my purpose I prefer to define natural law as God's natural way of defining reality. Natural law establishes the standard or the measure of ethics in reality. Natural law tells us what we ought not to do and what we ought to do. When natural man makes a decision to act one way or the other, then his action reflects his morality. For instance when an unbeliever becomes angry with another person, what restrains the unbeliever from murder. God's law, from God's Word, states "do not murder" and yet the unbeliever does not have the Word of God, but does not murder. Why did he keep God's law? Why does the unbeliever not commit adultery, steal, lie, or covet, even though he does not have the word of God? There is an epistemological dimension to this whole debate. Knowledge is ultimately inseparable from reality. Then how does the unbeliever keep the law of God if he doesn't know the law of God? The answer must be that the law of God is a rational and complete system of natural laws implanted in the hearts of men. To say anything different is

---

[90] Thomas Aquinas, *Summa Theologicia*, 618.

to deny the clear teaching of Scripture. The law of God was naturally implanted in the heart of Adam and Eve, Cain and Abel, Noah and his sons, Abram, Joseph even before the law of God was written in stone. All these men of old depended on the law of God written in their hearts. Natural law was abundantly sufficient to condemn their sins and remind them of the excellent perfections of God's holiness and the need for salvation.

If the law of God was natural to Adam and his progeny, where did natural law come from? It comes from God. Man is in a state of moral dependency from the Independent Being that created him. It would be out of character for that Independent Being to allow the dependent being to self-destruct. If the Independent Being did not give the dependent being regulations to control his behavior, then the dependent being would not survive. To put it another way the dependent being would have no purpose for existence.

Now if you ask, "how did I arrive at that conclusion, I would say natural theology of course." We naturally know certain things about the nature and character of God. Dr. James Henley Thornwell said it best. "Natural theology is that knowledge of God and of human duty which is acquired from the light of nature, or from the principles of human reason, unassisted by a supernatural revelation"[91]   This great Southern Presbyterian theologian understands that ethics are "acquired from the light of nature." Let me quote from another of God's servants. "If the light of Natural Theology makes us certain of anything, it assures us of these two facts, that God is a righteous ruler, and that we are transgressors."[92] It seems that those Southern Presbyterian theologians thought carefully and critically about natural law as it is found in Romans 2:14,15.

If we know we are transgressors then we know we have violated the law of God. Even more significant is that all men know they have violated the law and they know it through the natural means God has appointed for all men or the supernatural means God has appointed for His people. The inspired apostle Paul said, "Gentiles, who do not have the law, by nature do the things in the law" (New King James Version, Romans 2: 14). The New American Standard translates it this way: "Gentiles who do not have the Law do instinctively the things of the law." The New English Bible translation is: "When Gentiles who do not possess the law carry out its precepts by the light of nature, then, although they have no law, they are their own law, for they display the effect of the law inscribed on their hearts."

---

[91] James Henley *Thornwell, Theological*, p. 31.
[92] R. L. Dabney, *The Practical Philosophy* (Harrisonburg, VA: Sprinkle Publications, 1984), p. 518.

The light of nature sounds so familiar and it should because it is found often in the *Westminster Confession of Faith*. The Westminster theologians were not afraid of natural theology or natural law as it should be obvious in their frequent use of "the light of nature." The following examples from the *Westminster Confession of Faith* speak for themselves:

- Chapter I, of the Holy Scriptures (1.1) "the light of nature manifests the goodness, wisdom and power of God."
- Chapter X, of Effectual Calling (10.4) - Men cannot be saved "be they ever so diligent to frame their lives according to the light of nature."
- Chapter XXI, of Religious Worship and the Sabbath Day (21.1) - "The light of nature showeth that there is a God, who hath lordship and sovereignty over all."
- Chapter XXI, of Religious Worship and the Sabbath Day (21.1) - "As it is of the law of nature, that, in general, a due proportion of time be set apart for the worship of God."

Natural law whether it is called the light of nature or the law of nature is found in Romans 2:14 when the apostle uses the word "nature." The Greek noun *phusis*, translated nature in the English text (Romans 2:14) describes a native condition. *Phusis* refers to a natural condition or to natural characteristics. In some early Greek writings *phusis* referred to the product of nature. When we speak of nature we speak of particular characteristics which are natural. For instance, within humanity the nature of the male is distinguished from that of the female.

When the apostle Paul used the words "by nature" it seems to me to be unnatural to say there is no natural law. When unbelievers do the things of the law by nature, it seems natural to call it natural law. Natural men fashion their moral lives according the natural law written in their hearts. Supernatural men, those human beings who are new creatures in Christ, also have the law of God before them by means of the Bible and they desire to live according to its dictates. Natural man does not desire to live according to God's law. Natural man keeps the law because of self-interest, not because he loves the law maker.

For some reason or the other Christians today want to place natural law and the moral law of God antithetical to each other. If they mean that God's law cannot exist apart from God, they are correct. As I've already stated, it is not conceivable that a dependent being can have existence, intelligence, or order without being under the absolute authority and power of an Independent Being.

We do know the Bible teaches some things are unnatural. "For this cause God gave them up unto vile affections: for even their women did change the natural use into that which is against nature" (Romans 1:26). It is against nature to do that which is against God's law. The only way to go against natural law is to suppress it, to which every man is endowed with the capability to suppress God's law to a greater or lesser degree. If they mean that God's law is not natural to the human race, as God has given it to the human race, the age-old question stares us in the face: how does man obtain the law? How do professing atheists keep the law?

The confusion and sometimes the contradiction are almost too much for the human mind. For instance, let me quote from the Westminster Theological Journal.

- "To be sure, Reformed theology opposes any and all forms of autonomous natural theology, including natural law. "
- "Morality is established directly by God through supernatural or special revelation."
- "Just as every individual knows the true God, though not savingly, each person has the things of the law written upon his/her heart (Rom 1:18-2:16)."[93]

Some theologians call natural law by the term natural morality. Playing word games will not resolve this difficult dispute. The Bible makes it very clear that the

---

[93] Mark Karlberg, "Covenant and Common Grace," *Westminster Theological Journal* 50 (Fall 1988) : 323-337.

unbelieving world (nations, notice the plural) has the moral law by nature.

In Romans chapter 2 verse 15 the English Bible (NKJV) states "They show the work of the law written in their hearts." The English word "show" is translated from the Greek word *endeiknumi* meaning to inform against another party. We are not exaggerating if we say it means "to prove." The action of the verb "show" or "prove" reflects an ongoing action. I should also mention that Paul's assertion reflects certainty in the factual assertion of his proof. It is so clear that Scripture teaches the moral law by nature is shown or proven in the lives of all people.

I find it interesting that Paul used the terminology "written" on their hearts. God wrote the law on the tablets prepared by Moses (Exodus 34:1 and 34:28). Now we must ask what it means that the law of God is written on the heart. The word heart in the New Testament might refer to the one of several things. It could refer to the soul of man, but the heart may also simply refer to one aspect of the soul, such as the mind or the emotions. One theologian says the "heart" is always in Scripture the source of the instinctive feelings from which those impulses go forth which govern the exercise of the understanding and will."[94]

---

[94] Frederick L. Godet, *Commentary on the Epistle to the Romans* (Grand Rapids, MI : Zondervan Publishing House, 1956), p. 124.

The soul of man is not an instinctive essence because God endows the souls of men with the power of reason. Man is fallen, a sinner and unable to please God, but man is still able to think and make decisions. It is not our rational inability that allows us to see our own ignorance and sinfulness. It is God's law written on the heart. As Dr. John Gerstner has so well said, "It is the moral, not the natural, image which was lost in the fall."[95] The heart of unbelieving man finds the moral law distasteful, but not because he does not know the law, but because his conscience and rational abilities still exist. Natural man has a natural law, but he hates the lawgiver. They hate God because of his perfect moral character.

That brings us to the work of the conscience. The Bible refers to the conscience "bearing witness" is an active force (Romans 2:15). Whether the conscience is conceptual or a component of the mind is a question for metaphysical inquiry. The mind and the conscience are not always the same thing in Scripture. Jonathan Edwards' comments on the conscience are worth mention.

> Conscience is a principle implanted in the heart of every man, and is as essential to his nature as the faculty of reason, for it is a natural and necessary attendant of that faculty. But the will of a wicked

---

[95] Gerstner, *Rational Biblical Theology*, Vol. 2, p. 352.

man is contrary to it, and inconsistent with it. They choose those things which they know to be evil, and ought not to be chosen; they choose that which their own reason tells them is unreasonable and vile, and unbecoming men, and justly provoking to their Maker, and contrary to the end for which they are made.[96]

The concept of self-awareness must be associated with the conscience.

We cannot separate "self-awareness" from the mind or the will. In Romans 2:15 the conscience indicates human responsibility associated with self-awareness. I've read one place or the other that "the conscience is the central self-awareness of the knowing mind and acting will."

The unbeliever's conscience bearing witness is not dissociated from "their thoughts accusing or else excusing them." The Greek word for "thoughts" is *logismos*. This word could legitimately be translated "reasoning." Apparently the conscience is influenced by the reasonings of the unregenerate unbeliever. Sometimes his conscience convicts him by the reasoning he employs in the process of carrying on some kind of intelligent process. There are other times that his conscience excuses him even when he is guilty of violating God's law. There is either a little

---

[96] Gerstner, *Rational Biblical Theology*, vol. 2, p. 245.

voice inside saying "what you're doing is bad" or it may say "what you're doing is good" even though in reality it is bad. For sure, human beings should not trust their conscience, because it is still under the influence of sin. If Christians understand that "the law of God which we call the moral law is nothing else than a testimony of natural law and of that conscience which God has engraved upon the minds of men,"[97] then natural law and the moral law are the same.

For sure when Christians talk about natural law, they are not talking about any aspect of human law devised apart from the word of God. Natural law comes from God's moral law and God's moral law is found in the Word of God.

The main objection to natural law is that man is a fallen creature. Since unregenerate man is only interested in self-interest, he is unable in any moral sense to obey God. I say that when a sinner obeys the law of God he does so because of his natural ability and not his moral ability. As a result God is displeased with any obedience on the part of the unregenerate man.

I want to remind you that the law of God written on the hearts of all men evidences itself in one of two different ways.

---

[97] John Calvin, *The Institutes of the Christian Religion*, 2 vols. (Philadelphia, PA: The Westminster Press, 1960), vol. 2, p.1504.

The conscience bearing witness
The thoughts (reasoning) accusing or defending

Since the conscience is the central self-awareness of the knowing mind and the acting will, the conscience has its own distinct function. The question is whether or not the conscience can err? Will the conscience always act on the side of truth? Or does the conscience concern itself with moral decisions? We have to go back to the fall. What happened when Eve and Adam ate of the forbidden fruit? The *Westminster Confession of Faith* consults the full counsel of God to answer the question. "By this sin they fell from their original righteousness, and communion with God, and so became dead in sin, and wholly defiled in all the faculties and parts of soul and body."[98]

What does it mean that men are defiled in all the faculties and parts of soul and body? The Westminster Confession of Faith answers that question with precision and biblical accuracy. "After God had made all other creatures, he created man, male and female, with reasonable and immortal souls, endued with knowledge, righteousness, and true holiness after his own image having the law of God written in their hearts."[99]

---

[98] *Westminster Confession of Faith*, 6.2.
[99] Ibid., 4.2.

Reason and morality are two essential aspects of the soul? Reason is concerned with the powers of the mind. The only question that remains is whether or not the mind was destroyed at the fall. Theologians use the terminology "noetic effect of sin" in reference to this question. To put it another way, how was the mind affected by the fall of man? We know for certain that the fall did not destroy the mind. The mind was defiled, but not destroyed. The ability to function, make decisions and recognize God's law written on the heart is related to the works of the conscience. Now we come back to the question, can the conscience err? Will the conscience always act on the side of truth? Or does the conscience concern itself with moral decisions?

Since the conscience is the central self-awareness of the knowing sinful mind it may or may not be trusted to comprehend the truth of God's law. The will chooses according to its inclination at the time. The mind understands and the will acts according to its nature. The law of God written on the hearts of all men obligates them to an absolute and ultimate authority.

I hope you can better see the necessity for teaching the biblical views of that we call natural law. Without natural law Paul could not have said and would not have said "therefore you are without excuse" (Romans 2:1). Paul's arguments are inescapably before us and we should present this inescapable truth to all men. This biblical doctrine will be a great help in defending the faith before unbelievers.

The Jews have the law written on tablets; The Gentiles have the law written on their hearts. Both are without excuse. Whether it is the law of nature or the law of the stones, or the eternal law, or the moral law, their consciences bear witness and their reasoning powers condemn those who are without Jesus Christ.

The approaching judgment of Christ must also be considered in light of this discussion on natural law. The apostle Paul remembers the Psalmist said, "for he knoweth the secrets of the heart." Jesus said: "These people draw near to Me with their mouth And honor Me with their lips, But their heart is far from Me. And in vain they worship Me, teaching as doctrines the commandments of men" (Matthew 15:8). There are people who enumerate some of the good things that such and such person has done. Outward works are not a measure of how well one keeps the law of God. Outward works are spurious, occasional and even they are often tainted with obvious evil intentions. External works, pomp, pageantry and false proclamations will not deceive the righteous eye of God. These things will never replace truth and reality. Truth is the prerequisite for Christian apologetics. Reality will not hide from truth. All men, both Jews and Gentiles, will be judged by Christ as Christ himself said, "For not even the Father judges anyone, but He has given all judgment to the Son" (John 5:22).

Yes, Jesus Christ will judge the living and the dead to see if they have any interest in Him. If Christ does not find that righteousness, they shall perish and be condemned to everlasting punishment in Hell. This final judgment will reveal the secrets, motives, and principles that govern men. Everything will be brought to light. Nothing will be hidden because natural law demands that the wisest heathen be judged by the law of God.

The Herald of Truth

The herald of truth will defend the faith and announce the good news of God's saving grace. The apostle Paul was a master apologist. He was trained to defend the truth and he had plenty of occasions to practice his apologetical skills. Paul lived in a religious world that worshipped many false gods. His apologetic was to defend the truth of Christianity in the face of false religions. Paul's Christian apology prefaced the evangelistic message of the gospel. Defending the faith will not change the heart of an unbeliever. The evangelistic message will not change the heart of an unbeliever. Only the Holy Spirit is able to change the heart so the unbeliever will be able to believe the truth of God's saving grace. Every Christian world and life view ought to include both apologetics and evangelism.

The word evangelism comes from a Greek word that means "good message." The "ism" suffix denotes an action, practice, or literally a way of life. Like apologetics, evangelism ought to be a way of life for all Christians. It is the duty and should be the desire of every child of the kingdom of Jesus Christ to announce the goods news of the kingdom.

Evangelism is different from apologetics in that evangelism necessarily involves the kingdom concept. The kingdom of God is both dynamic and God-centered. God's supernatural power expressed by His dynamic working in time and space brings evangelism in everyday life. Evangelism is accompanied by God expressing His self-existent and creative rule over all. The kingdom is spiritual and eternal, but it is also material and temporal. American Christians do not understand the kingdom concept because the democratization of Christianity has created a world view known as individualism. Jesus is the King of kings; therefore He is the King of salvation. If Jesus is the king of salvation, He is the king of evangelism.

The law of accountability ought to be taken into account when Christians make their apology or announce the good news of the kingdom of Jesus Christ. "For everyone to whom much is given, from him much will be required; and to whom much has been committed, of him they will ask the more" (Luke 12:48). The King of kings endows Christians with abilities, gifts, and privileges to defend the truth of the kingdom and announce the gospel of the kingdom. The more opportunity king Jesus gives you to announce the gospel, the more you will be held accountable.

King Jesus said "go and make disciples" (Matthew 28:19). He did not say to make converts. The Holy Spirit is very capable of changing the heart so that one is able to believe the gospel of God's saving grace. (See Acts 16:14.)

Christians are the instruments or means that God uses to instruct the truth of God for the purpose of conversion.

When evangelism replaces apologetics, eventually revivalism will replace evangelism. The history of the Protestant church in North America is replete with examples. Although I have lost the source I retained a comment made by a Scottish minister in the latter part of the 19th century.

> It will be a sad day for our country if the men, who luxuriate in the excitement of man-made revivals, shall with their one-sided views of truth, which have ever been the germs of serious errors, their lack of spiritual discernment, and their superficial experience, become the leaders of the religious thought and the conductors of religious movements. They may be successful in galvanizing, by a succession of sensational shocks, a multitude of dead, till they seem to be alive, and they raise them from their crypts, to take a place amidst the living in the house of the Lord; but far better would it be to leave the dead in the place of the dead, and to prophesy to them there, till the living God himself shall quicken them, For death will soon resume its sway.

The leaders of religious thought are first in line to teach new converts the principles of apologetics and evangelism.

They will be held accountable for their doctrine and practice of apologetics and evangelism.

Are Christians running from the ungodly culture or are they embracing it? It may sound contradictory, but Christians are doing both. They tend to retreat from culture when culture begins to ask those difficult questions about what they believe and their religion. However they embrace the things that culture has to offer to make them successful and happy. Would you like to attack culture rather than retreat? Then ask your pastor, elder, deacon, or some other church leader to disciple the church with biblical principles of apologetics and evangelism. Follow in the foot steps of the apostle Paul and defend the faith with your Christian apology.

About the Author

Martin Murphy has a B.A. in Bible from Columbia International University and Master of Divinity from Reformed Theological Seminary. Martin spent nearly thirty years in the class room, the pulpit, the lectern, the study, and the library. He now devotes most of his time consolidating academic and practical gains by writing books. He and his wife Mary live in Dothan, Alabama. He is the author of numerous Christian books.

The Church: First Thirty Years, 344 pages, ISBN 9780985618179, $15.95. This book is an exposition of the Book of Acts. It will help Christians understand the purpose, mission, and ministry of the church.

The Dominant Culture: Living in the Promised Land, 172 pages, ISBN 970991481118, $11.95. This book examines the culture of Israel during the period of the Judges. It explains how worldviews influence the church and it reveals biblical principles to help Christians learn how to live in the culture.

The Essence of Christian Doctrine, 200 pages, ISBN 9780984570812, $12.95. This book was written so that pastors and laymen would have a quick reference to major biblical doctrines. Dr. Steve Brown says it was written, "with clarity and power about the verities of the Christian faith and in a way that makes a difference in how we live."

Return to the Lord, 130 pages, ISBN 9780984570805, $8.95. This book is an exposition of Hosea. The prophet speaks a message of repentance and hope. Hosea's prophetic message to Old Testament and New Testament congregations is, "you have broken God's covenant; return to the Lord." Dr. Richard Pratt said, "We need more correct and practical instruction in the prophetic books, and you have given us just that."

Theological Terms in Layman Language, 130 pages, ISBN 9780985618155, $8.95. This book was written so that simple words like faith or not so simple words like aseity are explained in plain language. Theological Terms in Layman Language is easy to read and designed for people who want a brief definition for theological terms. The terms are in layman friendly language.

Brief Study of the Ten Commandments, 164 pages, 9780991481163, $10.95. This book will help Christians discover or re-discover the meaning of the Ten Commandments.

The Present Truth, 164 pages, ISBN 9780983244172, $8.95. Each chapter examines a topic relative to the Christian life. Topics such as church, sin, anger, marriage, education and more.

Doctrine of Sound Words: Summary of Christian Theology, 423 pages, ISBN 9780991481125, $16.95. This is a book of Christian doctrine in topical format. It covers a wide range of theological topics such as, the triune God, creation, providence, sin, justification, repentance, Christian liberty, free will, marriage and divorce, Christian fellowship, et al). There are thirty three topics beginning with "Holy Scriptures" and ending with "The Last Judgment." It is a systematic theology for laymen based on the full counsel of God.

Friendship: The Joy of Relationships, ISBN 9780986405518, 48 pages, $6.49. This is the kind of book that friends give each other and share the principles with each other. If friends do not feel comfortable sharing these relationship principles with each other, the friendship may not really exist. Friendship involves a relationship of distinction. It is a relationship that respects the dignity of another person. The Bible teaches a different version of what it means to be a friend than the popular culture teaches. There are many occasions when friends say they are friends, but they are not friends. "Even my own familiar friend in whom I trusted, who ate my bread, has lifted up his heel against me" (Psalm 41:9). A true friend will endure and sacrifice for a friend. "A friend loves at all times" (Proverbs 17:7) and "there is a friend who sticks closer than a brother" (Proverbs 18:24).

Ultimate Authority for the Soul, ISBN 9780986405501, 151 pages, $9.99. What is the ultimate authority for human beings? This book examines that question and concludes that every rational being has some recognition of God as the ultimate authority. Although God is the ultimate authority, He confers His authority by means of the Word of God. The author examines Psalm 119 to build a defense for the ultimate authority for the soul. Although this book was written for Christians, the author builds the case that authority is a principle necessary to maintain sanity and order in the family, the church and civil society. The Word of God connects the soul with reality.